VEGETARIAN KIDNEY

DISEASE COOKBOOK

Nourishing recipes for a healthier, meat-free life

Emily Smith

TABLE OF CONTENTS

INTRODUCTION 7

Health Benefits of a Vegetarian Diet 9

Importance of Protein in a Vegetarian Diet 11

Chapter 1: Breakfast Recipes 14

Veggie Omelet 14

Avocado Toast with Tomatoes 16

Tofu Scramble... 17

Cinnamon Apple Oatmeal... 18

Smoothie Bowl... 19

Chickpea Flour Pancakes.. 20

Sweet Potato and Black Bean Breakfast Bowl 22

Quinoa Breakfast Bowl.. 23

Chapter 2: Appetizers and Snacks 25

Hummus with Veggies... 25

Sweet Potato Fries.. 26

Roasted Garlic and White Bean Dip 27

Baked Kale Chips 29

Fruit Skewers with Yogurt Dip...................................... 30

Edamame... 31

Caprese Salad Skewers 32

Spicy Roasted Chickpeas... 33

Roasted Red Pepper Hummus 34

Zucchini Fries 35

Chapter 3: Salads... 37

Spinach and Quinoa Salad with Roasted Vegetables ... 37

Mediterranean Chickpea Salad 39

Roasted Beet and Goat Cheese Salad 40

Caesar Salad with Avocado Dressing............................ 41

Fruit Salad with Honey Lime Dressing 43

Chapter 4: Soups.. 45

Tomato Basil Soup... 45

Minestrone Soup 47

Lentil Soup... 48

Butternut Squash Soup... 50

Potato Leek Soup 52

Chapter 5: Main Dishes 54

Vegetable Stir Fry with Brown Rice............................ 54

Baked Tofu with Roasted Vegetables......................... 56

Lentil and Vegetable Shepherd's Pie 58

Vegetable Curry... 60

Black Bean Enchiladas 61

Stuffed Portobello Mushrooms................................ 63

Vegetable Stir Fry.. 65

Eggplant Parmesan.. 67

Cauliflower Curry.. 68

Chapter 6: Side Dishes 71

Roasted Brussel Sprouts with Garlic and Lemon 71

Sauteed Kale with Almonds.................................. 72

Grilled Asparagus with Balsamic Glaze..................... 74

Quinoa and Vegetable Salad................................. 75

Sweet Potato Fries.. 77

Chapter 7: Desserts 79

Fruit Salad with Mint....................................... 79

Chocolate Avocado Pudding.. 80

Blueberry Oat Bars 81

Berry Chia Pudding.. 83

Peanut Butter Banana Ice Cream 85

CONCLUSION 87

INTRODUCTION

Once upon a time, there was an aspiring author who dreamed of writing a book that would change people's lives. She had a passion for cooking and had spent years experimenting with various recipes, perfecting them to suit her taste buds. But there was one particular area she felt compelled to explore, and that was creating recipes for people with kidney disease who followed a vegetarian diet.

The author had seen firsthand the impact of kidney disease on her own family members and close friends. She had watched them struggle with dietary restrictions and the difficulty of finding delicious, kidney-friendly meals that fit their vegetarian lifestyle. It was then that she realized that there was a gap in the market that needed to be filled, and she knew she was the person to do it.

With a fire in her belly and a pen in her hand, the author set out to write a book that would not only provide people with kidney disease who followed a vegetarian diet with delicious recipes but would also educate them on how to manage their dietary requirements. She spent months researching the subject, speaking to doctors, and learning everything there was to know about kidney disease and how a vegetarian diet could benefit those with the condition.

The author found that a vegetarian diet could be an excellent choice for people with kidney disease, as it provided them with the right balance of nutrients while also reducing their risk of developing other chronic illnesses such as heart disease and diabetes. But despite this, she found that many people were still unsure about how to make a vegetarian diet work for them, particularly when it came to getting enough protein.

So, armed with her research and her passion for cooking, the author set out to create a cookbook that would help people with kidney disease who followed a vegetarian diet to not only meet their dietary requirements but to also enjoy delicious and satisfying meals. She poured her heart and soul into the project, testing and retesting recipes until she was satisfied that they were both kidney-friendly and delicious.

As she wrote, the author imagined the joy that her book would bring to people's lives. She could see the smiles on their faces as they sat down to enjoy a meal with their families and loved ones, knowing that they were not only eating something delicious but also something that was good for their health.

And now, after months of hard work and dedication, the author's dream has become a reality. This book, her book, is now ready to be shared with the world, and she hopes that it will bring joy, health, and happiness to everyone who reads it.

Health Benefits of a Vegetarian Diet

A vegetarian diet is characterized by the exclusion of meat, poultry, and fish from one's diet. Instead, vegetarians rely on a wide variety of plant-based foods, such as fruits, vegetables, whole grains, legumes, and nuts, to meet their nutritional needs.

Research has shown that a vegetarian diet can offer numerous health benefits. One of the main advantages of a vegetarian diet is its association with a lower risk of chronic diseases such as heart disease, diabetes, and certain types of cancer.

Heart Disease

A vegetarian diet has been found to be effective in reducing the risk of heart disease. According to a 2019 study published in the Journal of the American Heart Association, vegetarians had a 25% lower risk of developing heart disease compared to non-vegetarians. The study also found that vegetarians had lower levels of cholesterol, blood pressure, and body mass index (BMI), which are all risk factors for heart disease.

Diabetes

Type 2 diabetes is a chronic condition characterized by high blood sugar levels. Research has shown that a vegetarian diet can help reduce the risk of developing type 2 diabetes. A 2015 study published in the PLOS Medicine journal found that vegetarians had a 34% lower risk of developing type 2 diabetes compared to non-vegetarians. The study also found that the longer a person followed a vegetarian diet, the lower their risk of developing diabetes.

Cancer

A vegetarian diet has been found to have a protective effect against certain types of cancer. A 2014 study published in the JNCI Cancer Spectrum journal found that vegetarians had a lower risk of developing colon cancer compared to non-vegetarians. The study also found that vegetarians had a lower risk of developing other types of cancer, including breast cancer and prostate cancer.

Importance of Protein in a Vegetarian Diet

One of the main concerns about a vegetarian diet is the potential for inadequate protein intake. Protein is an essential nutrient that is needed for the growth and repair of tissues in the body. It is also important for the production of enzymes, hormones, and other substances that help the body function properly.

Although it is true that meat is a rich source of protein, there are many plant-based foods that are also good sources of protein. Vegetarians can meet their protein needs by incorporating a variety of protein-rich foods into their diet.

Protein-Rich Vegetarian Foods
- Legumes

Legumes are an excellent source of protein, and they are a staple food in many vegetarian diets. Lentils, chickpeas, black beans, and kidney beans are all high in protein and can be used in a variety of dishes, such as soups, stews, and salads.

- Nuts and Seeds

Nuts and seeds are another good source of protein. Almonds, walnuts, cashews, and pumpkin seeds are all high in protein and can be added to breakfast cereals, salads, and trail mixes.

- Whole Grains

Whole grains such as quinoa, brown rice, and oats are also good sources of protein. These grains can be used in a variety of dishes, such as stir-fries, salads, and casseroles.

- Dairy Products

Dairy products such as milk, cheese, and yogurt are also good sources of protein. However, it is important to note that not all vegetarians consume dairy products, as some follow a vegan diet.

- Soy Products

Soy products such as tofu, tempeh, and edamame are excellent sources of protein. These foods are also rich in other nutrients such as iron and calcium, making them a healthy addition to a vegetarian diet.

Chapter 1: Breakfast Recipes

Breakfast is considered the most important meal of the day, and for good reason. It provides your body with the fuel it needs to get through the day, and can set the tone for the rest of your meals. This is especially true for those with kidney disease, who need to carefully consider the ingredients and nutritional value of their meals. In this chapter, we will explore a variety of vegetarian breakfast recipes that are kidney-friendly and delicious.

Veggie Omelet

Ingredients:

- 2 large eggs
- 1 tablespoon olive oil
- 1/4 cup chopped onion
- 1/4 cup chopped green bell pepper
- 1/4 cup chopped mushroom
- 1/4 cup shredded cheddar cheese
- Salt and pepper to taste

Instructions:

1. In a small bowl, beat the eggs with salt and pepper.
2. Heat the olive oil in a non-stick skillet over medium heat.
3. Add the onion, bell pepper, and mushroom, and sauté until tender.
4. Pour the beaten eggs over the sautéed vegetables, and let cook until the bottom is set.
5. Use a spatula to fold the omelet in half, and sprinkle the shredded cheese on top.
6. Cover the skillet with a lid and let cook for another 1-2 minutes, until the cheese is melted.
7. Serve hot.

This omelet is high in protein, and the vegetables add fiber, vitamins, and minerals. It is important to use a non-stick skillet to avoid adding extra fat to the dish.

Avocado Toast with Tomatoes

Ingredients:

- 1 slice whole wheat bread
- 1/2 avocado, mashed
- 1/2 cup cherry tomatoes, halved
- Salt and pepper to taste

Instructions:

1. Toast the bread.
2. Spread the mashed avocado on top of the toast.
3. Add the halved cherry tomatoes.
4. Season with salt and pepper to taste.
5. Serve immediately.

This breakfast is high in healthy fats, fiber, and vitamins. Whole wheat bread is a good source of complex carbohydrates, which provide sustained energy throughout the day.

Tofu Scramble

Ingredients:

- 1/2 block of firm tofu
- 1 tablespoon olive oil
- 1/4 cup chopped onion
- 1/4 cup chopped green bell pepper
- 1/4 cup chopped mushroom
- 1/4 teaspoon turmeric
- Salt and pepper to taste

Instructions:

1. Drain the tofu and press with paper towels to remove excess water.
2. Crumble the tofu into small pieces with a fork.
3. Heat the olive oil in a non-stick skillet over medium heat.
4. Add the onion, bell pepper, and mushroom, and sauté until tender.
5. Add the crumbled tofu to the skillet, and sprinkle with turmeric, salt, and pepper.

6. Use a spatula to mix everything together, and let cook until heated through.

7. Serve hot.

This dish is a great alternative to scrambled eggs, as tofu provides a good source of protein without the cholesterol found in eggs.

Cinnamon Apple Oatmeal

Ingredients:

- 1/2 cup rolled oats
- 1 cup water
- 1/2 cup unsweetened applesauce
- 1/2 teaspoon cinnamon
- 1 tablespoon chopped nuts (optional)

Instructions:

1. Combine the rolled oats and water in a microwave-safe bowl.

2. Microwave on high for 1-2 minutes, until the oats are cooked.
3. Stir in the applesauce and cinnamon.
4. Top with chopped nuts, if desired.

This breakfast is a hearty and satisfying option, with fiber from the oats and applesauce, and healthy fats from the nuts. Cinnamon is a delicious and warming spice that is also believed to have anti-inflammatory properties.

Smoothie Bowl

Ingredients:

- 1 cup frozen mixed berries
- 1/2 banana
- 1/2 cup unsweetened almond milk
- 1 tablespoon chia seeds
- 1 tablespoon honey
- Toppings: sliced banana, chopped nuts, shredded coconut, etc.

Instructions:

1. Combine the frozen mixed berries, banana, almond milk, chia seeds, and honey in a blender.
2. Blend until smooth.
3. Pour the mixture into a bowl.
4. Top with sliced banana, chopped nuts, shredded coconut, or any other toppings of your choice.
5. Serve immediately.

Smoothie bowls are a popular and delicious breakfast option, and can be customized with different fruits and toppings. Chia seeds add fiber and healthy omega-3 fatty acids, while the almond milk provides calcium without the phosphorus found in dairy milk.

Chickpea Flour Pancakes

Ingredients:

- 1 cup chickpea flour
- 1/4 teaspoon baking powder
- 1/4 teaspoon salt

- 1/4 teaspoon cumin
- 1/4 teaspoon turmeric
- 1/4 teaspoon paprika
- 3/4 cup water
- 1 tablespoon olive oil
- Toppings: salsa, sliced avocado, chopped cilantro, etc.

Instructions:

1. In a medium bowl, whisk together the chickpea flour, baking powder, salt, cumin, turmeric, and paprika.
2. Add the water and olive oil, and whisk until well combined.
3. Heat a non-stick skillet over medium heat.
4. Pour 1/4 cup of the batter onto the skillet for each pancake.
5. Cook until the edges start to dry and the bottom is golden brown, then flip and cook for another 1-2 minutes.
6. Serve hot with your favorite toppings.

These pancakes are high in protein and fiber, and the chickpea flour provides a good source of iron.

Sweet Potato and Black Bean Breakfast Bowl

Ingredients:

- 1 small sweet potato, cubed
- 1/2 cup black beans, drained and rinsed
- 1/4 teaspoon cumin
- Salt and pepper to taste
- 1 tablespoon olive oil
- 1 large egg
- Toppings: salsa, sliced avocado, chopped cilantro, etc.

Instructions:

1. Preheat the oven to 400°F (200°C).
2. Toss the sweet potato cubes with the black beans, cumin, salt, pepper, and olive oil.

3. Spread the mixture on a baking sheet and roast for 20-25 minutes, until tender and golden brown.

4. In a non-stick skillet, fry the egg to your liking.

5. Serve the roasted sweet potato and black bean mixture in a bowl, topped with the fried egg and your favorite toppings.

This breakfast bowl is high in protein, fiber, and vitamins, and the sweet potato provides a good source of potassium.

Quinoa Breakfast Bowl

Ingredients:

- 1 cup cooked quinoa
- 1/2 cup unsweetened almond milk
- 1/2 teaspoon cinnamon
- 1 tablespoon honey
- 1/2 cup sliced strawberries
- 1/4 cup chopped walnuts

Instructions:

1. In a medium saucepan, combine the cooked quinoa, almond milk, cinnamon, and honey.
2. Heat over medium heat, stirring occasionally, until heated through.
3. Divide the quinoa mixture between two bowls.
4. Top each bowl with sliced strawberries and chopped walnuts.
5. Serve hot.

This breakfast bowl is high in protein, fiber, and healthy fats, and the quinoa provides a good source of iron.

These vegetarian breakfast recipes are not only delicious but also kidney-friendly. They provide a variety of nutrients, including protein, fiber, healthy fats, and vitamins, while being low in sodium, potassium, and phosphorus. Eating a nutritious breakfast can help you maintain stable blood sugar levels, feel fuller for longer, and start your day off on the right foot. Try incorporating these recipes into your morning routine and enjoy a tasty and healthy breakfast!

Chapter 2: Appetizers and Snacks

When it comes to snacking, it's easy to reach for pre-packaged and processed options. However, these snacks are often high in sodium, sugar, and unhealthy fats, which can be detrimental to our health. That's why we've put together a list of vegetarian and kidney-friendly snack options that are both tasty and nutritious.

Hummus with Veggies

Hummus is a classic Middle Eastern dip made from chickpeas, tahini, lemon juice, and garlic. It's high in protein and fiber, making it a great option for kidney patients. You can serve hummus with a variety of veggies, such as carrots, cucumbers, bell peppers, and cherry tomatoes. Not only is it a tasty and healthy snack, but it's also easy to make at home.

To make hummus, you'll need:

- 1 can of chickpeas (drained and rinsed)
- 1/4 cup of tahini

- 2 cloves of garlic
- Juice of 1 lemon
- 2 tablespoons of olive oil
- Salt and pepper to taste

To prepare:

1. Combine all ingredients in a food processor or blender.
2. Blend until smooth and creamy.
3. Adjust seasoning to taste.
4. Serve with veggies for dipping.

Sweet Potato Fries

French fries are a popular snack option, but they're often deep-fried and high in unhealthy fats. Sweet potato fries are a healthier alternative, as they're baked instead of fried and contain more fiber and nutrients than regular potatoes. They're also a great source of vitamin A, which is important for kidney function.

To make sweet potato fries, you'll need:

- 2 sweet potatoes
- 2 tablespoons of olive oil
- Salt and pepper to taste

To prepare:

1. Preheat oven to 425°F.
2. Cut sweet potatoes into thin, even slices.
3. Toss sweet potatoes in olive oil and season with salt and pepper.
4. Spread sweet potatoes out in a single layer on a baking sheet.
5. Bake for 20-25 minutes, flipping halfway through, until fries are crispy and golden brown.

Roasted Garlic and White Bean Dip

This dip is a great alternative to hummus, as it's also high in protein and fiber. White beans are a good source of iron, which is important for kidney function. The roasted garlic adds a rich and savory flavor to the dip.

To make roasted garlic and white bean dip, you'll need:

- 1 can of white beans (drained and rinsed)
- 1 head of garlic
- 2 tablespoons of olive oil
- Juice of 1 lemon
- Salt and pepper to taste

To prepare:

1. Preheat oven to 400°F.
2. Cut the top off the head of garlic to expose the cloves.
3. Drizzle with 1 tablespoon of olive oil and wrap in foil.
4. Roast garlic for 30-40 minutes, until cloves are soft and caramelized.
5. Squeeze roasted garlic cloves out of their skins and add to a food processor.
6. Add white beans, lemon juice, remaining olive oil, salt, and pepper to the food processor.
7. Blend until smooth and creamy.
8. Adjust seasoning to taste.
9. Serve with veggies or crackers for dipping.

Baked Kale Chips

Kale chips are a healthy and crunchy snack option that's easy to make at home. Kale is high in antioxidants and vitamin K, which is important for bone health. Baking kale chips instead of frying them makes them a healthier alternative to potato chips.

To make baked kale chips, you'll need:

- 1 bunch of kale
- 2 tablespoons of olive oil
- Salt and pepper to taste

To prepare:

1. Preheat oven to 350°F.
2. Wash kale and pat dry with a paper towel.
3. Remove kale leaves from the stems and tear into bite-sized pieces.
4. Toss kale with olive oil and season with salt and pepper.
5. Spread kale out in a single layer on a baking sheet.

6. Bake for 10-15 minutes, until kale is crispy and lightly browned.

Fruit Skewers with Yogurt Dip

Fruit skewers are a refreshing and healthy snack option that's easy to make. You can use a variety of fruits, such as strawberries, pineapple, mango, and kiwi. The yogurt dip adds a creamy and tangy flavor to the skewers.

To make fruit skewers with yogurt dip, you'll need:

- Assorted fruits, cut into bite-sized pieces
- Wooden skewers
- 1 cup of plain Greek yogurt
- 1 tablespoon of honey
- 1 teaspoon of vanilla extract

To prepare:

1. Thread fruit onto skewers.
2. In a separate bowl, whisk together yogurt, honey, and vanilla extract.

3. Serve fruit skewers with yogurt dip.

Edamame

Edamame is a popular Japanese snack that's high in protein and fiber. It's a good source of iron and vitamin C, which is important for kidney function. You can buy frozen edamame in the supermarket and boil it at home.

To make edamame, you'll need:

- Frozen edamame
- Salt to taste

To prepare:

1. Bring a pot of water to a boil.
2. Add edamame and boil for 3-5 minutes, until beans are tender.
3. Drain edamame and sprinkle with salt.

Caprese Salad Skewers

Caprese salad skewers are a delicious and easy snack to make. They're also a great way to incorporate fresh vegetables and herbs into your diet. This recipe is kidney-friendly and perfect for summer barbecues or parties.

To make caprese salad skewers, you'll need:

- Cherry tomatoes
- Fresh mozzarella cheese, cut into small cubes
- Fresh basil leaves
- Wooden skewers
- Balsamic vinegar
- Salt and pepper to taste

To prepare:

1. Thread one cherry tomato, one cube of mozzarella, and one basil leaf onto a skewer.
2. Repeat until skewer is full.
3. Drizzle with balsamic vinegar and season with salt and pepper.

Spicy Roasted Chickpeas

Spicy roasted chickpeas are a great alternative to traditional potato chips. They're high in protein and fiber and have a delicious crunch. This recipe is easy to make and can be customized with your favorite spices.

To make spicy roasted chickpeas, you'll need:

- 1 can of chickpeas, drained and rinsed
- 1 tablespoon of olive oil
- 1 teaspoon of cumin
- 1/2 teaspoon of paprika
- 1/2 teaspoon of garlic powder
- Salt and pepper to taste

To prepare:

1. Preheat oven to 400°F.
2. Toss chickpeas with olive oil and spices.
3. Spread chickpeas out in a single layer on a baking sheet.

4. Bake for 20-30 minutes, until chickpeas are crispy and lightly browned.
5. Season with salt and pepper.

Roasted Red Pepper Hummus

Roasted red pepper hummus is a delicious and kidney-friendly snack option. It's high in protein and fiber and can be served with a variety of vegetables or crackers. This recipe is easy to make and can be stored in the refrigerator for up to a week.

To make roasted red pepper hummus, you'll need:

- 1 can of chickpeas, drained and rinsed
- 1 roasted red pepper
- 2 cloves of garlic
- 2 tablespoons of tahini
- 2 tablespoons of lemon juice
- 1/4 cup of olive oil
- Salt and pepper to taste

To prepare:

1. In a food processor, blend chickpeas, roasted red pepper, garlic, tahini, and lemon juice.
2. Gradually add olive oil until desired consistency is reached.
3. Season with salt and pepper.

Zucchini Fries

Zucchini fries are a healthy and kidney-friendly alternative to traditional french fries. They're low in sodium and high in fiber and vitamin C. This recipe is easy to make and can be served as a snack or side dish.

To make zucchini fries, you'll need:

- 2 zucchinis, cut into fry-shaped pieces
- 1/4 cup of breadcrumbs
- 1/4 cup of parmesan cheese
- 1/2 teaspoon of garlic powder
- 1/2 teaspoon of paprika
- Salt and pepper to taste

- 1 egg, beaten

To prepare:

1. Preheat oven to 425°F.
2. In a shallow dish, mix together breadcrumbs, parmesan cheese, garlic powder, paprika, salt, and pepper.
3. Dip zucchini pieces into the beaten egg, then coat in the breadcrumb mixture.
4. Place zucchini fries on a baking sheet and bake for 15-20 minutes, until golden brown and crispy.

Chapter 3: Salads

Salads are a great way to incorporate a variety of vegetables and fruits into your diet. They can be simple or complex, but they always offer a refreshing and healthy meal option. In this chapter, we will explore some delicious vegetarian salad recipes that are perfect for those with kidney disease.

Spinach and Quinoa Salad with Roasted Vegetables

This salad is packed with nutrition and flavor. Spinach is an excellent source of vitamins and minerals, while quinoa offers protein and fiber. Roasted vegetables add depth and texture to the dish.

Ingredients:

- 2 cups baby spinach
- 1 cup cooked quinoa
- 1 cup roasted vegetables (such as bell peppers, zucchini, and eggplant)

- 1/4 cup crumbled feta cheese
- 2 tbsp chopped walnuts
- 2 tbsp balsamic vinaigrette

Instructions:

1. Preheat oven to 375°F.
2. Cut bell peppers, zucchini, and eggplant into bite-sized pieces and place on a baking sheet.
3. Drizzle with olive oil and season with salt and pepper.
4. Roast for 20-25 minutes or until tender and lightly browned.
5. In a large bowl, combine spinach, quinoa, roasted vegetables, feta cheese, and walnuts.
6. Drizzle with balsamic vinaigrette and toss to combine.
7. Serve immediately.

Mediterranean Chickpea Salad

This salad is inspired by the flavors of the Mediterranean and is loaded with protein, fiber, and healthy fats. It's perfect for a light lunch or a side dish for dinner.

Ingredients:

- 2 cups cooked chickpeas
- 1 cup chopped cucumber
- 1 cup cherry tomatoes, halved
- 1/4 cup chopped red onion
- 1/4 cup chopped kalamata olives
- 1/4 cup crumbled feta cheese
- 2 tbsp chopped fresh parsley
- 2 tbsp lemon juice
- 1 tbsp olive oil
- 1 clove garlic, minced
- Salt and pepper, to taste

Instructions:

1. In a large bowl, combine chickpeas, cucumber, cherry tomatoes, red onion, kalamata olives, feta cheese, and parsley.
2. In a small bowl, whisk together lemon juice, olive oil, garlic, salt, and pepper.
3. Pour dressing over salad and toss to combine.
4. Serve immediately or refrigerate until ready to serve.

Roasted Beet and Goat Cheese Salad

Beets are a nutrient powerhouse, loaded with antioxidants and vitamins. In this salad, they are paired with creamy goat cheese and crunchy almonds for a delicious and satisfying meal.

Ingredients:

- 2 cups baby spinach
- 2 medium beets, roasted and chopped
- 1/4 cup crumbled goat cheese

- 2 tbsp chopped almonds
- 2 tbsp balsamic vinaigrette

Instructions:

1. Preheat oven to 375°F.
2. Wash and trim beets, then wrap them in foil and place on a baking sheet.
3. Roast for 45-60 minutes, or until tender.
4. Remove from oven, let cool, and peel off skin.
5. Chop beets into bite-sized pieces and set aside.
6. In a large bowl, combine baby spinach, chopped beets, crumbled goat cheese, and chopped almonds.
7. Drizzle with balsamic vinaigrette and toss to combine.
8. Serve immediately.

Caesar Salad with Avocado Dressing

This Caesar salad is a healthier version of the classic, with a creamy avocado dressing that is packed with flavor and nutrition

Ingredients:

- 2 cups chopped romaine lettuce
- 1/4 cup grated parmesan cheese
- 1/4 cup croutons
- 1 avocado, pitted and peeled
- 1 garlic clove, minced
- 1 tbsp lemon juice
- 1 tbsp olive oil
- Salt and pepper, to taste

Instructions:

1. In a large bowl, combine chopped romaine lettuce, grated parmesan cheese, and croutons.
2. In a blender or food processor, combine avocado, garlic, lemon juice, olive oil, salt, and pepper.
3. Blend until smooth and creamy.
4. Pour dressing over salad and toss to combine.
5. Serve immediately.

Fruit Salad with Honey Lime Dressing

This refreshing fruit salad is a great way to satisfy your sweet tooth while also getting a dose of vitamins and antioxidants. The honey lime dressing adds a tangy sweetness that pairs perfectly with the fresh fruit.

Ingredients:

- 2 cups mixed fruit (such as strawberries, blueberries, kiwi, and mango)
- 2 tbsp chopped fresh mint
- 1 tbsp honey
- 1 tbsp lime juice
- 1 tsp lime zest

Instructions:

1. Wash and chop fruit into bite-sized pieces and place in a large bowl.
2. In a small bowl, whisk together chopped fresh mint, honey, lime juice, and lime zest.

3. Pour dressing over fruit and toss to combine.

4. Serve immediately or refrigerate until ready to serve.

Salads are a great way to incorporate a variety of vegetables, fruits, and healthy ingredients into your diet. With the recipes in this chapter, you can enjoy delicious and healthy salad options that are perfect for those with kidney disease. Whether you're looking for a simple side dish or a complete meal, these salad recipes are sure to please your taste buds and nourish your body.

Chapter 4: Soups

Soup is a hearty, comforting dish that can be enjoyed year-round. Whether you're looking to warm up on a cold winter day or seeking a light, refreshing meal in the summer, soups offer a variety of options to satisfy any craving. In this chapter, we will explore five delicious soup recipes that are both vegetarian and kidney-friendly.

Tomato Basil Soup

Tomato basil soup is a classic recipe that never goes out of style. It's simple to make and full of flavor. This recipe is also low in sodium, making it a great option for those with kidney disease.

Ingredients:

- 2 tbsp olive oil
- 1 onion, chopped
- 3 cloves garlic, minced
- 2 cans (28 oz each) whole peeled tomatoes

- 4 cups low-sodium vegetable broth
- 1/4 cup chopped fresh basil
- 1/2 tsp salt
- 1/4 tsp black pepper

Instructions:

1. Heat the olive oil in a large pot over medium heat.
2. Add the onion and garlic and sauté for 5-7 minutes, until soft and fragrant.
3. Add the tomatoes (including the juice from the can) and vegetable broth. Bring to a boil.
4. Reduce the heat to low and simmer for 20-25 minutes.
5. Use an immersion blender to blend the soup until smooth.
6. Add the chopped basil, salt, and black pepper. Stir to combine.
7. Serve hot.

Minestrone Soup

Minestrone soup is a hearty, vegetable-based soup that is perfect for a satisfying meal. This recipe is loaded with kidney-friendly vegetables and is a great source of protein thanks to the addition of cannellini beans.

Ingredients:

- 2 tbsp olive oil
- 1 onion, chopped
- 3 cloves garlic, minced
- 2 stalks celery, chopped
- 2 carrots, chopped
- 1 zucchini, chopped
- 1 can (28 oz) diced tomatoes
- 4 cups low-sodium vegetable broth
- 1 can (15 oz) cannellini beans, drained and rinsed
- 1/2 cup uncooked small pasta
- 1/4 cup chopped fresh parsley
- 1/2 tsp salt
- 1/4 tsp black pepper

Instructions:

1. Heat the olive oil in a large pot over medium heat.
2. Add the onion and garlic and sauté for 5-7 minutes, until soft and fragrant.
3. Add the celery, carrots, and zucchini. Sauté for 5-7 minutes, until the vegetables are tender.
4. Add the diced tomatoes (including the juice from the can), vegetable broth, and cannellini beans. Bring to a boil.
5. Reduce the heat to low and simmer for 20-25 minutes.
6. Add the pasta and simmer for an additional 10-12 minutes, until the pasta is cooked.
7. Add the chopped parsley, salt, and black pepper. Stir to combine.
8. Serve hot.

Lentil Soup

Lentil soup is a delicious and nutritious meal that is perfect for a cold winter day. This recipe is rich in fiber, protein, and iron, making it an excellent choice for those with kidney disease.

Ingredients:

- 2 tbsp olive oil
- 1 onion, chopped
- 3 cloves garlic, minced
- 1 carrot, chopped
- 1 stalk celery, chopped
- 1 cup dried brown lentils, rinsed and drained
- 4 cups low-sodium vegetable broth
- 1 bay leaf
- 1/2 tsp salt
- 1/4 tsp black pepper
- 2 tbsp chopped fresh parsley

Instructions:

1. Heat the olive oil in a large pot over medium heat.
2. Add the onion and garlic and sauté for 5-7 minutes, until soft and fragrant.

3. Add the carrot and celery and sauté for an additional 5-7 minutes, until the vegetables are tender.

4. Add the lentils, vegetable broth, bay leaf, salt, and black pepper. Bring to a boil.

5. Reduce the heat to low and simmer for 30-40 minutes, until the lentils are tender.

6. Remove the bay leaf and discard.

7. Use an immersion blender to blend the soup until smooth.

8. Add the chopped parsley and stir to combine.

9. Serve hot.

Butternut Squash Soup

Butternut squash soup is a delicious and comforting soup that is perfect for a chilly evening. This recipe is low in sodium and high in vitamin A, making it a great choice for those with kidney disease.

Ingredients:

- 2 tbsp olive oil
- 1 onion, chopped

- 3 cloves garlic, minced
- 1 butternut squash, peeled, seeded, and chopped
- 4 cups low-sodium vegetable broth
- 1/2 tsp ground cinnamon
- 1/2 tsp ground nutmeg
- 1/2 tsp salt
- 1/4 tsp black pepper
- 1/4 cup plain Greek yogurt

Instructions:

1. Heat the olive oil in a large pot over medium heat.
2. Add the onion and garlic and sauté for 5-7 minutes, until soft and fragrant.
3. Add the butternut squash and sauté for an additional 5-7 minutes, until the squash is tender.
4. Add the vegetable broth, cinnamon, nutmeg, salt, and black pepper. Bring to a boil.
5. Reduce the heat to low and simmer for 20-25 minutes, until the squash is very tender.
6. Use an immersion blender to blend the soup until smooth.

7. Stir in the Greek yogurt until well combined.

8. Serve hot.

Potato Leek Soup

Potato leek soup is a rich and creamy soup that is perfect for a cozy night in. This recipe is low in sodium and high in potassium, making it a great option for those with kidney disease.

Ingredients:

- 2 tbsp unsalted butter
- 2 leeks, white and light green parts only, sliced
- 3 cloves garlic, minced
- 3 potatoes, peeled and chopped
- 4 cups low-sodium vegetable broth
- 1/2 cup heavy cream
- 1/2 tsp salt
- 1/4 tsp black pepper

Instructions:

1. Melt the butter in a large pot over medium heat.
2. Add the leeks and garlic and sauté for 5-7 minutes, until soft and fragrant.
3. Add the potatoes and vegetable broth. Bring to a boil.
4. Reduce the heat to low and simmer for 20-25 minutes, until the potatoes are very tender.
5. Use an immersion blender to blend the soup until smooth.
6. Stir in the heavy cream, salt, and black pepper until well combined.
7. Serve hot.

Soups are a great way to get a variety of nutrients in one meal. They are easy to prepare, delicious, and can be customized to your taste preferences. The soup recipes in this chapter are perfect for vegetarians with kidney disease, as they are low in sodium, high in fiber, and packed with nutritious ingredients. So next time you're in the mood for something warm and comforting, try one of these delicious soup recipes.

Chapter 5: Main Dishes

Main dishes are the backbone of any vegetarian meal. They provide the bulk of the nutrients and proteins that your body needs to function properly. In this chapter, we will explore some delicious and healthy main dish recipes that are perfect for anyone following a vegetarian diet.

Vegetable Stir Fry with Brown Rice

Stir fry is a classic dish that is perfect for any vegetarian meal. It is quick and easy to prepare, and it can be made with a variety of vegetables. For this recipe, we will be using brown rice instead of white rice to make it even healthier.

Ingredients:

- 2 cups brown rice
- 2 tbsp olive oil
- 1 onion, chopped
- 2 cloves garlic, minced
- 1 red bell pepper, sliced

- 1 green bell pepper, sliced
- 1 cup snow peas
- 1 cup broccoli florets
- 1 cup sliced mushrooms
- 2 tbsp soy sauce
- 1 tbsp honey
- 1 tbsp cornstarch
- 1/4 cup water
- Salt and pepper to taste

Instructions:

1. Cook brown rice according to package instructions.
2. Heat olive oil in a large skillet over medium-high heat.
3. Add onion and garlic and cook until onion is translucent.
4. Add red and green bell peppers, snow peas, broccoli, and mushrooms. Cook for 5-7 minutes or until vegetables are tender.
5. In a small bowl, whisk together soy sauce, honey, cornstarch, and water.

6. Add the sauce to the skillet and stir until vegetables are coated.

7. Season with salt and pepper to taste.

8. Serve stir fry over cooked brown rice.

Baked Tofu with Roasted Vegetables

Tofu is a great source of protein for vegetarians. It is also very versatile and can be used in a variety of dishes. In this recipe, we will be baking tofu with roasted vegetables for a healthy and delicious main dish.

Ingredients:

- 1 block of firm tofu
- 2 tbsp olive oil
- 1 onion, chopped
- 2 cloves garlic, minced
- 2 carrots, sliced
- 2 zucchinis, sliced
- 1 red bell pepper, sliced
- 1 yellow bell pepper, sliced

- 2 tbsp balsamic vinegar
- Salt and pepper to taste

Instructions:

1. Preheat oven to 400°F.
2. Drain tofu and press with a paper towel to remove excess water. Cut tofu into cubes.
3. In a large bowl, toss tofu with 1 tbsp of olive oil, salt, and pepper.
4. Spread tofu cubes on a baking sheet and bake for 20-25 minutes or until golden brown.
5. Meanwhile, heat 1 tbsp of olive oil in a large skillet over medium-high heat.
6. Add onion and garlic and cook until onion is translucent.
7. Add carrots, zucchinis, red and yellow bell peppers. Cook for 5-7 minutes or until vegetables are tender.
8. Add balsamic vinegar to the skillet and stir until vegetables are coated.
9. Season with salt and pepper to taste.

10. Serve roasted vegetables with baked tofu cubes on top.

Lentil and Vegetable Shepherd's Pie

Shepherd's pie is a classic comfort food that is perfect for a vegetarian meal. In this recipe, we will be using lentils instead of meat for a healthy and delicious twist on this traditional dish.

Ingredients:

- 2 cups cooked lentils
- 2 tbsp olive oil
- 1 onion, chopped
- 2 cloves garlic, minced
- 2 carrots, diced
- 2 celery stalks, diced
- 1 cup frozen peas
- 1 cup vegetable broth
- 1 tsp thyme
- Salt and pepper to taste
- 4 cups mashed potatoes

Instructions:

1. Preheat oven to 375°F.
2. In a large skillet, heat olive oil over medium heat.
3. Add onion and garlic and cook until onion is translucent.
4. Add carrots and celery and cook for 5-7 minutes or until vegetables are tender.
5. Add cooked lentils, frozen peas, vegetable broth, thyme, salt, and pepper. Stir well and let simmer for 10 minutes.
6. Pour lentil and vegetable mixture into a large baking dish.
7. Spread mashed potatoes evenly over the top of the mixture.
8. Bake in the oven for 25-30 minutes or until the top is golden brown.
9. Let cool for a few minutes before serving.

Vegetable Curry

Curry is a flavorful and aromatic dish that is perfect for a vegetarian meal. It is made with a variety of vegetables and spices, making it both healthy and delicious.

Ingredients:

- 2 tbsp olive oil
- 1 onion, chopped
- 2 cloves garlic, minced
- 1 tbsp grated ginger
- 2 tbsp curry powder
- 1 tsp ground cumin
- 1 tsp ground coriander
- 1 sweet potato, peeled and diced
- 2 carrots, diced
- 1 red bell pepper, sliced
- 1 zucchini, sliced
- 1 can chickpeas, drained and rinsed
- 1 can diced tomatoes
- 1 cup vegetable broth
- Salt and pepper to taste

Instructions:

1. Heat olive oil in a large pot over medium heat.
2. Add onion and garlic and cook until onion is translucent.
3. Add grated ginger, curry powder, cumin, and coriander. Cook for 1-2 minutes or until fragrant.
4. Add sweet potato, carrots, red bell pepper, and zucchini. Cook for 5-7 minutes or until vegetables are tender.
5. Add chickpeas, diced tomatoes, and vegetable broth. Stir well and bring to a boil.
6. Reduce heat and let simmer for 20-25 minutes or until vegetables are fully cooked.
7. Season with salt and pepper to taste.
8. Serve curry over cooked rice or with naan bread.

Black Bean Enchiladas

These enchiladas are a hearty and flavorful vegetarian meal that's easy to make and perfect for weeknight dinners.

Ingredients:

- 1 tbsp olive oil
- 1 onion, chopped
- 2 cloves garlic, minced
- 1 red bell pepper, chopped
- 1 can black beans, drained and rinsed
- 1 cup cooked corn
- 1 can diced tomatoes with green chilies
- 1 tsp chili powder
- 1 tsp ground cumin
- Salt and pepper to taste
- 8-10 corn tortillas
- 1 cup shredded cheddar cheese

Instructions:

1. Preheat oven to 350°F.
2. Heat olive oil in a large skillet over medium heat.
3. Add onion and garlic and cook until onion is translucent.

4. Add red bell pepper and cook for 5-7 minutes or until tender.

5. Add black beans, corn, diced tomatoes, chili powder, cumin, salt, and pepper. Stir well and let simmer for 10 minutes.

6. Spread a thin layer of the bean mixture on the bottom of a 9x13 inch baking dish.

7. Warm tortillas in the microwave or on a skillet until pliable.

8. Spoon some of the bean mixture onto each tortilla and roll up tightly.

9. Place the rolled-up tortillas in the baking dish, seam side down.

10. Cover with remaining bean mixture and sprinkle shredded cheese on top.

11. Bake in the oven for 25-30 minutes or until cheese is melted and bubbly.

Stuffed Portobello Mushrooms

These stuffed Portobello mushrooms make an elegant and satisfying vegetarian meal that's perfect for special occasions or dinner parties.

Ingredients:

- 4 large Portobello mushrooms
- 2 tbsp olive oil
- 1 onion, chopped
- 2 cloves garlic, minced
- 1 cup cooked quinoa
- 1 cup chopped spinach
- 1/2 cup crumbled feta cheese
- 1/4 cup chopped fresh parsley
- Salt and pepper to taste

Instructions:

1. Preheat oven to 375°F.
2. Remove stems from mushrooms and scrape out the gills with a spoon.
3. Brush mushroom caps with olive oil and place them on a baking sheet.
4. Heat olive oil in a large skillet over medium heat.
5. Add onion and garlic and cook until onion is translucent.

6. Add cooked quinoa, chopped spinach, feta cheese, parsley, salt, and pepper. Stir well and let cook for a few minutes.

7. Spoon the quinoa mixture into each mushroom cap, pressing down firmly.

8. Bake in the oven for 25-30 minutes or until mushrooms are tender and filling is hot.

Vegetable Stir Fry

Stir fry is a quick and easy vegetarian meal that's perfect for busy weeknights. This recipe uses a variety of colorful vegetables and flavorful sauce for a tasty and healthy meal.

Ingredients:

- 2 tbsp olive oil
- 1 onion, sliced
- 2 cloves garlic, minced
- 1 red bell pepper, sliced
- 1 yellow bell pepper, sliced
- 1 cup sliced mushrooms
- 1 cup snow peas

- 1/2 cup chopped green onions
- 1/4 cup soy sauce
- 2 tbsp honey
- 2 tsp cornstarch
- 1 tsp grated ginger

Instructions:

1. Heat olive oil in a large skillet or wok over high heat.
2. Add onion and garlic and stir fry for 1-2 minutes.
3. Add red and yellow bell peppers, mushrooms, and snow peas. Stir fry for 3-4 minutes or until vegetables are tender-crisp.
4. In a small bowl, whisk together soy sauce, honey, cornstarch, and grated ginger.
5. Pour the sauce over the vegetables and stir to coat evenly.
6. Cook for 1-2 minutes or until sauce has thickened.
7. Serve hot, garnished with chopped green onions.

Eggplant Parmesan

This classic Italian dish is traditionally made with breaded and fried eggplant, but this recipe uses a healthier baked version that's just as delicious.

Ingredients:

- 2 large eggplants, sliced into 1/2 inch rounds
- 1 cup all-purpose flour
- 3 eggs, beaten
- 2 cups seasoned breadcrumbs
- 1/4 cup grated Parmesan cheese
- 1 jar marinara sauce
- 2 cups shredded mozzarella cheese

Instructions:

1. Preheat oven to 375°F.
2. Place flour, beaten eggs, and breadcrumbs in three separate shallow dishes.
3. Dip eggplant slices into flour, then eggs, then breadcrumbs, shaking off excess.

4. Place breaded eggplant slices on a baking sheet and bake for 20-25 minutes or until golden brown.

5. Spread a thin layer of marinara sauce in the bottom of a 9x13 inch baking dish.

6. Arrange a layer of baked eggplant slices on top of the sauce.

7. Sprinkle grated Parmesan cheese on top of the eggplant.

8. Repeat layers of sauce, eggplant, and Parmesan until all ingredients are used up.

9. Top with shredded mozzarella cheese.

10. Bake in the oven for 25-30 minutes or until cheese is melted and bubbly.

Cauliflower Curry

This fragrant and spicy curry is made with cauliflower and chickpeas for a hearty and flavorful vegetarian meal that's perfect for chilly nights.

Ingredients:

- 1 tbsp olive oil

- 1 onion, chopped
- 2 cloves garlic, minced
- 1 head cauliflower, cut into small florets
- 1 can chickpeas, drained and rinsed
- 1 can diced tomatoes
- 1 can coconut milk
- 2 tbsp curry powder
- 1 tsp ground cumin
- 1/2 tsp ground turmeric
- Salt and pepper to taste
- Chopped fresh cilantro for garnish

Instructions:

1. Heat olive oil in a large pot over medium heat.
2. Add onion and garlic and cook until onion is translucent.
3. Add cauliflower florets and chickpeas, and stir well to coat with the onion and garlic mixture.
4. Add diced tomatoes, coconut milk, curry powder, cumin, turmeric, salt, and pepper.
5. Stir well and bring to a simmer.

6. Reduce heat to low and let simmer for 20-25 minutes or until cauliflower is tender.
7. Serve hot, garnished with chopped cilantro.

These vegetarian main dishes are sure to impress even the most ardent meat-lovers. They're packed with flavor, protein, and nutrients, and they're easy to prepare at home. Whether you're looking for a quick weeknight meal or an impressive dish to serve at your next dinner party, these recipes will not disappoint. Give them a try and see for yourself how delicious vegetarian cuisine can be!

Chapter 6: Side Dishes

When it comes to mealtime, side dishes are often overlooked, but they can make all the difference in turning a good meal into a great one. Whether you're serving a main dish or a simple salad, a well-crafted side dish can elevate the entire meal. In this chapter, we'll explore some delicious and nutritious vegetarian side dishes that are perfect for any occasion.

Roasted Brussel Sprouts with Garlic and Lemon

Ingredients:

- 1 lb. Brussel sprouts, trimmed and halved
- 3 cloves garlic, minced
- 1 lemon, juiced and zested
- 2 tbsp. olive oil
- Salt and pepper, to taste

Instructions:

1. Preheat your oven to 400°F (200°C).
2. In a large bowl, toss the Brussel sprouts with the garlic, lemon juice and zest, olive oil, salt, and pepper.
3. Spread the Brussel sprouts in a single layer on a baking sheet.
4. Roast in the preheated oven for 20-25 minutes, or until tender and lightly browned.

These roasted Brussel sprouts are packed with flavor and are a perfect side dish for any meal. The garlic and lemon add a bright and zesty flavor that balances the natural bitterness of the sprouts. Plus, roasting the sprouts in the oven brings out their natural sweetness and adds a delicious caramelized flavor.

Sauteed Kale with Almonds

Ingredients:

*   1 bunch kale, stems removed and leaves chopped

- 2 cloves garlic, minced
- 1/4 cup sliced almonds
- 2 tbsp. olive oil
- Salt and pepper, to taste

Instructions:

1. Heat the olive oil in a large skillet over medium-high heat.
2. Add the garlic and almonds and sauté for 1-2 minutes, or until the almonds are lightly toasted and the garlic is fragrant.
3. Add the chopped kale to the skillet and toss to combine with the garlic and almonds.
4. Cook for 5-7 minutes, or until the kale is tender and wilted.
5. Season with salt and pepper, to taste.

This sautéed kale with almonds is a simple and nutritious side dish that pairs well with any main dish. The almonds add a satisfying crunch, while the garlic and olive oil infuse the kale with a rich and savory flavor. Plus, kale is packed with vitamins and minerals, making it a great choice for a healthy and delicious side dish.

Grilled Asparagus with Balsamic Glaze

Ingredients:

- 1 lb. asparagus, trimmed
- 2 tbsp. olive oil
- Salt and pepper, to taste
- 1/4 cup balsamic vinegar
- 1 tbsp. honey

Instructions:

1. Preheat your grill to medium-high heat.
2. Toss the asparagus with olive oil, salt, and pepper.
3. Grill the asparagus for 4-5 minutes per side, or until tender and lightly charred.
4. While the asparagus is grilling, combine the balsamic vinegar and honey in a small saucepan over medium-high heat.

5. Bring the mixture to a boil and cook for 2-3 minutes, or until thickened and syrupy.

6. Drizzle the balsamic glaze over the grilled asparagus and serve immediately.

Grilled asparagus is a classic side dish that's perfect for summer cookouts or any time you want to add a touch of smoky flavor to your meal. The balsamic glaze adds a tangy sweetness that complements the earthy flavor of the asparagus perfectly. Plus, asparagus is packed with nutrients like fiber, folate, and vitamins A, C, and K, making it a healthy and delicious addition to any meal.

Quinoa and Vegetable Salad

Ingredients:

- 1 cup quinoa, rinsed and drained
- 2 cups vegetable broth or water
- 1 red bell pepper, diced
- 1 yellow bell pepper, diced
- 1 cucumber, diced
- 1/4 cup red onion, diced

- 1/4 cup fresh parsley, chopped
- 1/4 cup olive oil
- 2 tbsp. red wine vinegar
- 1 clove garlic, minced
- Salt and pepper, to taste

Instructions:

1. In a medium saucepan, combine the quinoa and vegetable broth or water.
2. Bring the mixture to a boil, then reduce the heat and simmer for 15-20 minutes, or until the quinoa is tender and the liquid is absorbed.
3. In a large bowl, combine the cooked quinoa, diced bell peppers, cucumber, red onion, and parsley.
4. In a small bowl, whisk together the olive oil, red wine vinegar, garlic, salt, and pepper.
5. Pour the dressing over the quinoa and vegetables and toss to combine.
6. Chill the salad in the refrigerator for at least 30 minutes before serving.

This quinoa and vegetable salad is a healthy and satisfying side dish that's perfect for picnics, potlucks, or any time you want a refreshing and nutritious side dish. Quinoa is a great source of plant-based protein and fiber, while the vegetables add color, flavor, and additional nutrients.

Sweet Potato Fries

Ingredients:

- 2 large sweet potatoes, peeled and cut into thin strips
- 2 tbsp. olive oil
- 1 tsp. paprika
- 1/2 tsp. garlic powder
- Salt and pepper, to taste

Instructions:

1. Preheat your oven to 425°F (220°C).
2. In a large bowl, toss the sweet potato fries with olive oil, paprika, garlic powder, salt, and pepper.
3. Spread the fries in a single layer on a baking sheet.

4. Roast in the preheated oven for 20-25 minutes, or until tender and crispy.

These sweet potato fries are a healthier alternative to traditional French fries, and they're just as tasty. The paprika and garlic powder add a savory and smoky flavor that complements the sweetness of the potatoes. Plus, sweet potatoes are a great source of vitamin A, fiber, and potassium, making them a nutritious addition to any meal.

Side dishes may not always be the star of the show, but they can make a big difference in the overall flavor and nutrition of your meal. These vegetarian side dishes are delicious, nutritious, and easy to prepare, making them perfect for any occasion. Whether you're looking for a refreshing salad, a savory sauté, or a crispy side dish, these recipes are sure to satisfy your taste buds and nourish your body. So why not give them a try and see how they can elevate your next meal?

Chapter 7: Desserts

After a satisfying meal, nothing beats a sweet treat to cap it off. However, people with kidney disease may find themselves avoiding traditional desserts because of their high potassium, phosphorus, and sodium content. But fear not, because with a little creativity and the right ingredients, there are still plenty of delicious desserts to indulge in. This chapter features some kidney-friendly dessert recipes that are not only tasty but also nutritious and easy to make.

Fruit Salad with Mint

Fruit salad is a classic dessert that is refreshing, light, and perfect for any occasion. This recipe features a variety of fresh fruits and a touch of mint for added flavor.

Ingredients:

- 2 cups diced watermelon
- 2 cups diced pineapple
- 2 cups diced strawberries

- 1 cup blueberries
- 1/4 cup chopped mint leaves
- 1 tablespoon honey (optional)

Instructions:

1. Combine all the fruits in a large mixing bowl.
2. Add the chopped mint leaves and honey, if using.
3. Toss everything together until the fruits are evenly coated with the mint and honey.
4. Chill the fruit salad in the refrigerator for at least 30 minutes before serving.

Chocolate Avocado Pudding

If you're a fan of chocolate, this avocado pudding recipe is a must-try. Avocado provides a creamy texture that complements the richness of chocolate, while also adding some healthy fats and fiber to the dish.

Ingredients:

- 2 ripe avocados

- 1/2 cup unsweetened cocoa powder
- 1/4 cup maple syrup
- 1/4 cup almond milk
- 1 teaspoon vanilla extract
- 1/4 teaspoon salt

Instructions:

1. Cut the avocados in half and remove the pits.
2. Scoop the avocado flesh into a food processor or blender.
3. Add the cocoa powder, maple syrup, almond milk, vanilla extract, and salt.
4. Blend everything together until smooth and creamy.
5. Transfer the pudding to a serving bowl or individual cups.
6. Chill the pudding in the refrigerator for at least 30 minutes before serving.

Blueberry Oat Bars

These blueberry oat bars are a wholesome and satisfying snack that can also double as a dessert. Oats are a good source of fiber, while blueberries provide antioxidants and flavor.

Ingredients:

- 1 cup rolled oats
- 1/2 cup oat flour
- 1/2 cup almond flour
- 1/4 cup chopped walnuts
- 1/4 cup coconut oil, melted
- 1/4 cup maple syrup
- 1 teaspoon vanilla extract
- 1/4 teaspoon salt
- 1 cup fresh or frozen blueberries

Instructions:

1. Preheat the oven to 350°F.
2. In a large mixing bowl, combine the oats, oat flour, almond flour, chopped walnuts, coconut oil, maple syrup, vanilla extract, and salt.

3. Mix everything together until a crumbly dough forms.

4. Line an 8-inch square baking dish with parchment paper.

5. Press half of the dough into the bottom of the baking dish, using your fingers or a flat spatula to create an even layer.

6. Spread the blueberries over the dough.

7. Cover the blueberries with the remaining dough, pressing it down gently.

8. Bake the oat bars in the preheated oven for 25-30 minutes, or until golden brown.

9. Let the bars cool completely in the baking dish before slicing into squares.

Berry Chia Pudding

Chia pudding is a versatile dessert that can be customized with different flavors and toppings. This berry chia pudding recipe is a perfect example, with the addition of mixed berries and coconut flakes for a tropical twist.

Ingredients:

- 1/4 cup chia seeds
- 1 cup unsweetened almond milk
- 1 tablespoon honey
- 1/2 teaspoon vanilla extract
- 1/2 cup mixed berries (such as raspberries, blackberries, and blueberries)
- 2 tablespoons unsweetened coconut flakes

Instructions:

1. In a mixing bowl, combine the chia seeds, almond milk, honey, and vanilla extract.
2. Whisk everything together until well combined.
3. Let the mixture sit for 10 minutes, then whisk again to break up any clumps of chia seeds.
4. Cover the bowl with plastic wrap and refrigerate for at least 4 hours or overnight.
5. When ready to serve, spoon the chia pudding into individual cups or bowls.

6. Top each serving with mixed berries and coconut flakes.

7. Enjoy!

Peanut Butter Banana Ice Cream

Who says you can't enjoy ice cream on a kidney-friendly diet? This peanut butter banana ice cream recipe is made with frozen bananas and peanut butter, making it a healthier alternative to traditional ice cream.

Ingredients:

- 4 ripe bananas, peeled and sliced
- 1/4 cup creamy peanut butter
- 1/4 cup unsweetened almond milk
- 1 teaspoon vanilla extract
- 1/4 teaspoon salt

Instructions:

1. Place the sliced bananas in a single layer on a baking sheet lined with parchment paper.

2. Freeze the bananas for at least 2 hours or until completely frozen.

3. In a food processor or blender, combine the frozen bananas, peanut butter, almond milk, vanilla extract, and salt.

4. Blend everything together until a smooth and creamy consistency is achieved.

5. Transfer the ice cream to a container and freeze for an additional 1-2 hours to firm up.

6. When ready to serve, let the ice cream sit at room temperature for 5-10 minutes to soften before scooping.

7. Enjoy!

Desserts don't have to be off-limits for people with kidney disease. By using kidney-friendly ingredients and being mindful of portion sizes, it's possible to enjoy sweet treats while still maintaining a healthy diet. These recipes are just a few examples of the many delicious and nutritious desserts that can be made without compromising kidney health. So go ahead and indulge in some guilt-free dessert!

CONCLUSION

As I come to the end of this book, I am filled with a sense of satisfaction and accomplishment. The Vegetarian Kidney Disease Cookbook was a labor of love, born out of my own personal struggle with kidney disease and the challenges of finding delicious and nutritious vegetarian meals that were safe for me to eat.

My hope is that this book has provided you with a wealth of information, resources, and most importantly, a collection of tasty and healthy recipes that will help you manage your kidney disease and improve your overall health and wellbeing.

Over the course of this book, I have emphasized the importance of adopting a vegetarian diet as a means of managing kidney disease. The benefits of a vegetarian diet are well-documented, and research has shown that vegetarians tend to have lower rates of chronic diseases such as heart disease, diabetes, and kidney disease.

One of the key benefits of a vegetarian diet for individuals with kidney disease is that it can help to reduce the load on the kidneys by limiting the intake of protein, sodium, and potassium. By focusing on plant-based proteins such as legumes, nuts, and seeds, and reducing or eliminating animal-based proteins, individuals with kidney disease can improve their kidney function and slow the progression of their disease.

In addition to protein, individuals with kidney disease must also be mindful of their intake of sodium and potassium. A high-sodium diet can contribute to high blood pressure and fluid retention, which can exacerbate kidney disease. Similarly, high levels of potassium in the blood can be dangerous for individuals with kidney disease, as the kidneys are responsible for filtering excess potassium from the body.

The recipes in this book are designed to be both nutritious and delicious, while also being safe for individuals with kidney disease to consume. I have included a variety of recipes for breakfast, appetizers and snacks, salads, soups, main dishes, side dishes, and desserts, so you can enjoy a wide range of flavors and textures.

I have also included tips and recommendations throughout the book for modifying recipes to fit your individual dietary needs. For example, if you need to limit your intake of potassium, you can substitute low-potassium vegetables in recipes that call for higher-potassium ingredients.

Throughout this book, I have emphasized the importance of working with a registered dietitian or other healthcare professional to develop a customized meal plan that meets your individual needs. While the recipes in this book are designed to be safe and healthy for individuals with kidney disease, it is important to work with a healthcare professional to ensure that your overall diet and lifestyle are optimized for managing your kidney disease.